Atkins Diet

Transform Your Life Through Atkins Diet - Tasty Recipes and Healthy Lifestyle

By Hannah Olson

Hannah Olson

paraphrase any part or the content within this book without the consent of the author or copyright owner. Legal action will be pursued if this is breached.

Disclaimer Notice:

Please note the information contained within this document is for educational and entertainment purposes only. Every attempt has been made to provide accurate, up to date and reliable complete information. No warranties of any kind are expressed or implied. Readers acknowledge that the author is not engaging in the rendering of legal, financial, medical or professional advice.

By reading this document, the reader agrees that under no circumstances are we responsible for any losses, direct or indirect, which are incurred as a result of the use of information contained within this document, including, but not limited to, —errors, omissions, or inaccuracies.

Table Of Contents

Hannah Olson

Introduction

Thank you for purchasing the book on Atkins Diet.

This diet is one of the best diets to have been created. Yes, this is not a diet that has existed for a long period, but a diet that has been created by Dr. Robert Atkins who is a cardiologist. This diet works on identifying the different types of food that will be able to match your metabolism. That sounds impossible does it not? But this is the main objective of the diet. When he had begun his research on the diet, Dr. Robert Atkins put his patients on a low sugar and carbohydrate diet. His theory that the human body needed either sugar or fat to survive was proved right through this diet!

The book covers the reasons why the Atkins diet was coined. It also explains to you the different benefits of this diet. Weight loss is not the only benefit of this diet, though that is the main aim. This diet has low amounts of carbohydrates and sugar, which ensures that you lose weight. This diet ensures that you lose weight faster when compared to a lot of other low – calorie diets.

There are different recipes in the book, which ensure that you have low amounts of sugar and carbohydrates. You will need some time to procure the food that is required to strictly follow this diet. This book makes your life easier! You have been provided with a list of grocery items. You can use this to gather all your ingredients for the first week. Try to ensure that you buy the groceries once every week. There may be times when you would want to stay off this diet. At such a time, try to motivate yourself. Do not give in to your emotions! You will live long and prosper if you follow this diet.

Thank you for purchasing the book. I hope you enjoy the recipes that have been provided in this book.

Chapter 1
The Atkins Diet

The Atkins diet, also known as the Atkins Nutritional Approach, was created by a Dr. Robert Atkins. He is a cardiologist who works in the United States of America. He had come across a diet in the Journal of the American Medical Association. He then devised another diet, which he tested on himself. He found himself losing weight. It was only after this that he began to use the diet on his patients.

But who is Dr. Robert Atkins?

About Dr. Robert Atkins

Dr. Robert Atkins had studied in the University of Michigan. He received his medical degree from the Cornell Medical College in the year 1955. He decided to specialize in cardiology and complementary medicine. During his practice he had authored many books of which Dr. Atkins'

Diet Revolution was his first. He later wrote many other books where he never moved away from his initial specifications for a diet. He always made sure that the diet that he devised was low on carbohydrates and low on sugar.

It was in April 2003 that Dr. Atkins passed away. He had slipped on ice on his way to work and hurt his head.

What is the Atkins Diet?

The main objective of the Atkins Diet is to ensure that a person's diet has a reduced intake of carbohydrates. The idea of the low carbohydrates diet comes majorly from the books that have been written by Dr. Robert Atkins. This diet has four phases, which have vitamin and mineral supplements. The diet has always been combined with exercise.

Dr. Atkins had said that human beings tend to ignore certain factors that are crucial to their eating habits. These factors are what make them fat. He said that the main reason why human beings put on weight is that they consume refined carbohydrates like sugar.

When you are on the Atkins diet, you will find that your body has begun to burn the excess fat that has been stored in your body instead of burning the glucose in your body to provide you with energy. This switch is called Ketosis. When the level of glucose is low in your body, the insulin levels also lower. This is when ketosis begins! This means that when you have very low levels of glucose in your body, your body looks at the fat reserves and burns the fat off in order to provide your body with fuel or energy.

Your body has low levels of glucose and insulin right before you eat. The minute you have finished your meal, the level of glucose rises in your body. This triggers the levels of insulin to rise. If you consume refined carbohydrates, you will realize that your blood stream is full of glucose.

There are other types of carbohydrates, called the 'good carbohydrates', which have a minimal impact on the level of glucose in your blood. These carbohydrates ensure that the fat that has been stored in the cells are transferred or moved to the blood during ketosis.

In Dr. Atkins' first book, he states that a diet, which has a low amount of refined carbohydrates in it, triggers the metabolism. Your body will begin to burn more calories than it would if you are on any other diet. It is during this process that your body starts to get rid of any calories that have been unused.

Dr. Atkins focuses majorly on a term 'Net Carbs'. This is the total carbohydrate that you have consumed minus the sugar alcohols and fiber. It has been found that the alcohols in sugar have absolutely no effect on the levels of sugar in your blood. Dr. Atkins has said that the best carbohydrates are the ones that have a low glycemic load. After conducting thorough research, Dr. Atkins has said that a person should ensure that his intake of saturated fats must be kept to a maximum of twenty percent of all the calories that he consumes.

Atkins has said that a patient suffering from Diabetes Type 2 or any other type of metabolic syndrome would find a subsequent decrease in the amount of sugar in his blood. He may also discover that he has no need for any medication. There are diabetics doctors who have stated that though the objective of the diet is vital for a patient with diabetes, the diet is not a very simple solution.

Chapter 2

The Four Phases of the diet

As mentioned above, there are four phases to this diet. This section explains these phases in detail.

Phase 1: Induction

You will need to ensure that the consumption of calories is reducing every day. Once your body has accepted the change, you will need to ensure that the amount of calories that you obtain through carbohydrates has been limited to only twenty grams per day. The main sources of such carbohydrates would be from your vegetables and salads, which are low on starch.

The first phase of this program is referred to as the induction phase, and the purpose of this phase is to get you started with the weight loss program. A very common misconception about the induction phase is that people mistake it for the whole program and not just the beginning of it. This induction phase in reality is all about getting your body to start its fat burning process. As you move along this diet you will realize that this diet lets you to gradually consume more Net Carbs while you continue to lose weight, keep your body energized and also keep a check on your appetite.

Objectives of the First Phase

Duration

You will need to let the induction phase go on for at least two weeks, but you can follow it for longer if you think that you have got to shed more weight or if you want to shed those extra pounds relatively faster. You can stay in this phase till you are just 15 pounds away from the goal you have set.

Purpose

The purpose of this diet is to help your body to shift to burning fat to produce energy instead of burning carbohydrates. This helps in kick starting the Atkins diet for weight loss.

Its goal

The goal of the first phase is to help you reduce the net carb intake to an average of 20 carbs per day. It cannot be less than a minimum of 18 grams of Net Carbs per day and this is the level at which burning of fat will take place.

FAQs about Phase 1 of the Atkins diet

Is Phase 1 compulsory?

No it isn't compulsory. In fact you can start at any of the three phases of the Atkins. If you want to shed just a few pounds up to 15 pounds then you can skip the Phase 1 and directly start Phase 2 and you can consume at least 25-30 grams of Net Carbs on a daily basis during the second phase. But if you were on the heavier side it would prove to be more beneficial if you start from the Phase 1, but then again you can always skip the first step. When you do this be prepared to be patient for longer because the task of shedding those extra kilos will take some extra time.

Is counting of carbs essential while following the meal plan?

No it isn't. However it is highly unlikely that you would follow the meal plan to the letter and it is also not possible to follow it strictly unless you consume all meals at home.

So, the best possible alternative would be to make use of a carb counter. Whatever the case might be, it is essential that you know how to count carbs, especially when you start adding some foods back. Carb counting just lets you double check and this improves your chances of success from the get go.

Are two snacks compulsory?

It isn't necessary that you consume two snacks every day. If you opt for having five small meals a day then you might not feel the need to consume snacks in between these meals. But whatever your meal plan is, you will need to ensure that the gap between two meals does not exceed four to six hours. If not a snack then you can always have a cup of a hot beverage or even a cup of broth if you prefer it.

What is water weight?

When you are following a diet, the first couple of pounds that you lose are water weight. Atkins in particular has diuretic effect. And this is the reason why it is essential that you consume a lot of water and keep your body properly hydrated. Eat all the foundation vegetables that you are required to consume along with the multivitamin supplements to replace all the lost electrolytes. When the excess fluid from your body is drained out even your electrolytes are washed out with it. Therefore, keep your body properly hydrated. Only after shedding this water weight will your body start burning off all the excess fat.

The amount of protein and fat that can be consumed

You cannot consume as much ever protein or fat that you want to consume. When you consume excess of protein or fat, then your body will start getting sluggish and interfere weight loss or create a calorie bomb that will mess with the weight loss program.

The amount of water to be consumed

Most of the people tend to be dehydrated most of the time. It is essential to drink a lot of water because it helps in getting rid of all the harmful toxins that get accumulated in our bodies during the course of day. Not just this but it also helps in fighting constipation and bad breath, provides lubrication for your joints and maintains your overall health. Keeping yourself hydrated will help in losing weight. You can also fulfill your daily water requirement by consuming small amounts of tea or any other beverage that hasn't been artificially sweetened or is pre-packed. Have some hot diluted soup or even vegetable broth if you feel like it.

Is it fine to consume bacon?

It is fine to consume bacon, but in moderation. If you are worried about all the sugar and maple the bacon or any pork products are cured in; then don't worry, these get burned off while cooking.

Is the carbohydrate count of all the vegetables the same after cooking them?

When you cook vegetables they get reduced or they become compact, especially leafy greens or cabbage. Carb count reflects the amount of veg you have cooked. When you slice or grate any vegetable it also compacts it more than slicing or chopping it. This affects the carb count.

Is it fine to consume deserts in Phase 1?

Yes it is safe, provided you have consumed the quota of foundation vegetables that is required by the diet and the net carb limit is not exceeded. One serving of desert should not exceed 3 grams of net carbs. The desert recipes provided in this book will help satiate your desert pangs without breaking any rules.

Indulging in more carbs by cutting carbs the next day

It is important you maintain a uniform level of carbohydrate consumption for your body if you don't want to mess with your blood sugar levels. An alteration in the range o f3 to 4 grams of Net Carbs between two days is fine, but not more than that. If you happened to overindulge yourself on one day, just return back to the prescribed intake the next day. Don't try to compensate it.

Is it okay to take a break from the diet on weekends?

If you do this, it means that your body will return to the primary blood sugar metabolism over the weekends. It takes your body a while to get acclimatized to kick-start the fat burning mechanism. And a constant shift in your diet will set back this process unnecessarily.

Does caffeine interfere with weight loss?

The initial guidelines for the Atkins diet required the individual to completely eliminate caffeine from their diet. But the rules have been liberalized, instead now they ask for reducing the consumption of caffeine.

How to move on to Phase?

After following Phase 1 of this diet for two weeks, it is time to decide whether you can move onto the next stage or stick to the current phase a while longer. Let us look at the ways in which you can move over to the next phase.

Fast track

If you are comfortable and motivated by the quick weight loss that you have experienced in the induction phase and are fine with the restriction on choices, then you can stay in Phase 1 for a while longer than the initial two weeks. You can make this process easier and can also set the stage for transition if you wish for it. Continue with the consumption of 20 grams of Net Carbs on a daily basis even after the initial two weeks and you can also add some nuts and seeds to your list of items fit for consumption. Nuts are low in carbs but are high in protein and fat.

To make things easier for you, you can swap 3 grams of Net Carbs you consume on a daily basis with alternate foods like a half a cup of green beans or even a small tomato or one and a half cups of mixed greens. Or even 3 grams of nuts or seeds will do, but ensure that you don't cut down on your foundation vegetables of 12 grams worth of Net Carbs on a daily basis. 3 grams worth of Net Carbs of seeds or nuts would roughly mean about 30 almonds, 3 tablespoons of macadamia nuts or even two tablespoons of peanut butter. If you like walnuts then about 24 walnuts will cover the net carb count. If you want to avoid overeating then you should probably sort out the required quantities beforehand itself.

You can move over to Phase 2 when you are 15 pounds away from your goal weight. This is the point when you have to shift yourself towards a more permanent way of healthy eating by introducing foods that are higher up on the Carb chart. You can top your salads with a few seeds or nuts as well, consume different seed and nut butters and nut flours that are available in supermarkets these days.

Go slow and steady

Instead of sticking with Phase 1 for a while longer, you can move over to Phase 2. Provided you are fine with the idea of losing weight gradually. You can do this by adding back 5 grams of Net Carbs back to your diet and also introduce foods that are higher up the carbohydrate chart, this allows you to feel energetic, in control of your appetite and lose weight as well. You will be able to understand the foods that are interfering with the weight loss program and get rid of them accordingly. You might find that you are comfortable with a low level of carb intake somewhere in between 25 and 30 grams of Net Carbs per day. This is not that different from the induction phase. You can start consuming certain seeds and nuts as well and also include berries, melons and cherries back into your diet. In the next stage you will be able to move onto more delicious foods such as Greek yogurt and even fresh soft cheeses. As the carb intake increases gradually, you can start adding back more delicious things back into your diet. It is essential to have a balanced diet irrespective of the stage, which you are at.

Phase 2: OWL (Ongoing Weight Loss)

It is essential that you add foods that are rich in nutrients and in fiber. These are the additional sources of carbohydrates. You will need to increase the quantity of these foods in your diet at the rate of twenty – five grams during the first week of this phase and 30 grams during the second week and the subsequent weeks till you find that there is no decrease in your weight. When you reach this stage, you will need to decrease the amount of carbohydrates by 5 grams every day till you find that you have begun to lose weight once again.

Overview of Phase 2

In Phase 2 of the Atkins diet you can start adding back different foods slowly and also move up the carb ladder. You can start consuming certain nuts, seeds, berries, melons, cottage cheese, yogurt and many more healthy foods. The basic objective of Phase 2 is to ensure that the momentum you have gained during the induction phase needs to be maintained.

Objectives

Duration

This phase can be followed till you are 10 pounds away from your goal and you can move onto Phase 3 sooner provide you are willing to slow down the process of weight loss.

Purpose

The purpose of the second phase is to get rid of the excess pounds and also find your personal carbohydrate balance.

Goals

You are going to start out at 25 grams of Net Crabs on a daily basis and then progressively increase you carb intake. This means you will have to slowly increase the variety of foods you are consuming and also include those foods that are higher up the carb ladder. You will need to figure out your ideal carb consumption and this will be affected by various factors including your gender, age, level of physical activity undertaken by you and many more.

FAQs about Phase 2

How to get back to your routine after an indiscretion

The first thing you will have to do is not beat yourself up for the "indiscretion". You need to realize that once in a while you might succumb to the urge of gorging on something you aren't supposed to. It is okay to do that. But don't continue with that trend for the whole day. Get back to your routine immediately; don't wait for the next day to start.

What is a carb creep?

You might unknowingly consume more carbs than you think you are when you start adding back foods to the list.

You need to keep a track of the portions you consume and also the carb intake. You shouldn't let the process of adding back foods mess with your weight loss program.

Reason for the return of cravings

Usually cravings for food tend to disappear after the first week of the induction phase, when your body shifts over to burning of fat. There are many reasons why your cravings might return. For women, their cravings tend to return right before their menstrual cycle. When the gap between meals is too long or adding certain foods like dairy and peanuts might also stimulate your cravings. Stress, decrease in blood sugar levels or even depression will increase your cravings for comfort food. Add a little more of fat to keep these cravings at bay. Fat will make you feel full and also help you fight off your cravings.

Is it compulsory to reintroduce all the foods acceptable under Phase 2?

Of course not! It is not essential that you need to consume all the acceptable foods. If you don't like chickpeas or even yogurt, you can skip it. You can eat what you like, as long as it falls within the acceptable range of foods. But do ensure that you aren't depriving your body of essential nutrients. That could be dangerous.

Reasons for erratic weight loss

The way your body functions, is much different than that of the next person. All you need to do is follow this diet faithfully and you will start shedding those extra kilos. If you toss in a bit of exercise then the weight loss will become easier. Taking weekly measurements will help you keep track of your progress. And if you have lost a few inches then the scale will catch up pretty soon.

Is it normal to regain some of the lost weight?

It is okay to gain back some weight. But by the end of this phase you would have lost weight and not gained any, provide you were faithful to the diet. You shouldn't weigh yourself on a daily basis. It so happens that your weight might vary by up to 5 pounds between two days and even the same day. As long as you are faithful to the diet, you will definitely lose some weight at the end of every week. If it doesn't happen, then you have probably retained some of the water weight or are probably constipated.

Shifting to Phase 3

Have you been losing weight steadily and are about 10 pounds away from your goal weight? Then it is time to move onto the third phase. Since you are only 10 pounds away from attaining your goal weight, you have got sufficient time to reintroduce more carbs into your meals.

Overview of Phase 3

You can get started with the third Phase of this diet provided that you are just 10 pounds from your goal weight, you can achieve this in Phase 3. This phase is designed to help you fine-tune your body to focus on maintaining the weight that you have lost. In this phase you will learn all about maintaining your weight and even shedding those few remaining pounds by raising your daily net carb intake.

Objectives

Duration

You can continue with this stage until you have achieved your weight loss goal and have been able to maintain that weight for at least 4 weeks.

Purpose

The purpose of this step is to get rid of those remaining extra pounds and also maintain the weight you have lost. In this process you will be able to identify your personal balance of carb intake. This phase is like a rehearsal for setting into the lifetime maintenance phase.

Goal

You will have to gradually increase the Net Carbs that you consume by increments of almost 5 to 10 grams. And keep reintroducing new foods that are rich in carbs. Provided that you are able to shed some weight and maintain it as well.

FAQs about Phase 3

Is it safe to consume a glass or two of wine?

It is all right to consume a glass of wine or two provided that this does not make you crave for carb rich snacks or pile on unnecessary weight that you have lost with great difficulty. If you observe any weight gain, then you should probably cut back on the wine.

What is the ideal weight?

The ideal weight will differ according to the height, weight, gender, age and a multitude of factors. So, there is no precise answer to this question. It all depends on your perception of the ideal weight you want to maintain.

How to tame cravings for anything sweet?

There are two ways in which you can control your urge for a sweet treat. Either fight it or indulge in it. If you are able to satiate your craving for something sweet by staying well within the daily net carb intake then you can satisfy your craving. If not then you will need to concentrate on eliminating such a craving.

Is it all right to consume deserts?

Yes it is. Go ahead and have some desert. You can look into the recipes that are mentioned in this book. Or one quick way to satiate this urge is by grabbing bowl of cream and berries. You can never go wrong with this. Provided you don't go over 9 grams of Net Carbs.

Transition into Phase 4

Now comes the big question, when do you move onto the next phase? If you can answer the following three questions with a confident yes, then it indeed is time to move onto the next stage.

a)   Have you reached your goal weight?

b)   Have you been able to maintain your weight at a constant level for at least 4 weeks?

c)   Do cravings and hunger no longer pose a problem?

Phase 4: Lifetime Maintenance

At this phase, you will have to begin to introduce a lot of different sources of carbohydrates. You will also have to monitor your weight to ensure that it does not increase. You should never let the sense of well–being go away. If you find that your weight has begun to increase, you can slowly begin to reduce two things – the amount of carbohydrates that you consume every day and any new carbohydrates that you may have introduced into your diet. According to Dr. Atkins, it is your lifestyle that will create a strong foundation for a lifetime with better health.

Overview of Phase 4

This is the last phase of the Atkins diet. Congratulations on making it this far. You have achieved your weight loss goal and now you have entered the stage of lifelong maintenance. This can be thought of as a lifestyle instead of a stage. In a general sense the foods that you consume during this stage are the ones that you have been consuming so far. You might have tried to reintroduce few foods earlier, but your efforts might have proved futile. Well, you can reintroduce those foods now. You can experiment with all these foods as long as you are close to your goal weight.

Objectives

Duration

This stage goes on forever. It is a lifestyle option.

Purpose

The purpose of this stage is to help you transition into a permanent way of eating healthy foods that will help you maintain your ideal weight.

Goal

The goal of this stage is to let you take the reins of your weight and adjust the intake of carbohydrates depending upon the tolerance of your body.

Have you gained a few pounds? But don't know how to deal with the situation? Maybe you have unknowingly overindulged yourself in foods you should have or some form of injury has prevented you from exercising regularly. Well, don't fret. You can reduce about 10 Net Crabs from your daily diet till you reach your goal weight again. Here are some options that you can eliminate if you want to return to your goal weight:

Half a banana, half a baked potato, half of a sweet potato, half a cup of cooked oatmeal, one cup of watermelon, two carrots, one slice of bread, some beets, rice, yogurt or chickpeas as well.

How to stay in control of your goal weight

Don't exceed to level of Net Carbs that you are consuming on a daily basis. Stay within the limit of carb tolerance (the level you discovered in Phase 3). Continue to consume at least 12-15 grams of daily quota of Net Carbs in the form of foundation vegetables. Consume a minimum of 4-6ounces of cooked protein in each meal. Two servings of fruit per day will do. Fat is your friend and essential for managing your weight, don't forget this. Carbs need to be combined with fat or protein or a combination of both if you want to keep a balanced level of blood sugar in your body. Keep drinking a lot of water, at least 8 four-ounce glasses per day and some more if you can. Depending upon your level of activity adjust the level of carbs you consume. Differentiate between hunger and a craving. Never let yourself put on more than 5 pounds of your goal weight. While adding new foods back into your diet add them one at a time and record how it affects your weight management process. Physical activity is a must. Nuts and cheese need to be divided into edible portions beforehand to avoid overeating. Read the labels of food products carefully. Beware of carb creep and also plan ahead for your meals. It is okay to take a break from the low carb lifestyle once in a while but don't make a habit of it.

The Principle of the Diet

The Atkins Diet works on four major principles. You will need to keep these in mind whenever you find yourself feeling low about not losing weight. The diet abides by these principles. You will find yourself losing weight if you follow this diet strictly. The four principles are:

1.   A person following this diet will definitely lose weight.

2.   You will definitely be able to maintain your weight after having lost it

3.   You will be able to ensure that you have good health

4.   You will set for yourself a strong foundation that will help you overcome and prevent any diseases.

Is the Atkins Diet effective?

It is true that any diet is effective when you stick to it. It is the same for the Atkins Diet. There have been researches conducted at the Stanford University. The conclusion of this research is that a person who followed the Atkins Diet has lower cholesterol levels, better blood pressure levels and has lost more weight when compared with the people following other diets.

When you stick to this diet, you will lose weight and will be able to keep it off. However, the problem is that it is difficult to stick to the diet. It was found that although ten percent of the adults were on the Atkins Diet during this decade, obesity and overweight continued to be the predominant disease in the country.

It was found that the craze to follow diets with low carbohydrates made no effect at all on the people, at least not on a national scale. It is true that low carbohydrate diets or diets with good carbohydrates in them work. It is the problem with the people. People continue to drop out of diets on account of being tired or bored.

There were many studies conducted year after year for a period of three years where it was found that a majority of the people who began the Atkins Diet did not continue it, not in the long term at least. It was found that people who stuck by the diet did fare better than most others for the reasons mentioned above.

Hannah Olson

Chapter 3

The Benefits Of The Atkins Diet

In the above chapter, you have learnt about the different principles and the phases of the Atkins Diet. From the principles you have learnt that this diet is good to ensure weight loss. But there are other benefits to this diet. This chapter covers those benefits in detail.

Epilepsy and other related diseases

There have been close to thirty-five studies that have been conducted between 2004 and 2014. These studies have stated that the Modified Atkins Diet has helped in reducing the symptoms of seizure disorders and epilepsy in children and adults. This study was encouraging for the children who have been diagnosed with childhood epilepsy and who have not been responding to the medication that was provided.

GERD

There have been other studies conducted that explain that a diet with low carbohydrates helps in alleviating acid reflux. Foods that have a high amount of caffeine in them or have high amounts of fats encourage acid reflux. There has been other research conducted that proves that the Atkins Diet which is a diet with low carbohydrates has a good effect on GERD.

Acne

There has been growing research that has been conducted on identifying the effect of the Atkins diet on the health of the skin. A review that was published in *'Skin Pharmacology and Physiology'* stated that a diet with low carbohydrates helped in reducing the amount of acne on the skin.

Heart Diseases

There have been twenty-one studies that have been conducted between the years 2002 and 2014, which try to identify the effect of a low carbohydrates diet on the heart. It was found that these diets help in decreasing the risk factor of heart diseases. They also help in lowering the risk of hypertension. It was found that these low carbohydrate diets have shown a decrease in the levels of cholesterol and also the levels of triglycerides. This helps in reducing the inflammation of glands thereby reducing the frequency of heart diseases.

Cancer

It has been seen that obesity is a factor that has been associated as a risk for some types of cancer. It, therefore, implies that if people follow a low carbohydrates diet which will help them lose and maintain their loss in weight, they will be able to prevent having some types of cancer.

PCOS

Polycystic Ovary Syndrome (PCOS) is one of the most common problems that is affecting women who are of the reproductive age. This problem is associated with obesity, hyperinsulinemia and the resistance of insulin. It has been found that diets with low carbohydrates have reduced the body's resistance towards insulin. It was also found that when women follow a diet with low carbohydrates, they are able to avoid the formation of a cyst in their ovaries.

Dementia

It has been found that a diet with a lot of calories in it is often associated with the increased risk of the impairment of the cognitive side of your mind. In the year 2012, it was shown in the Journal of Alzheimer's Disease that people who had a high carb diet faced a greater risk of being attacked by dementia. The Atkins Diet ensures that this impairment is reduced to a large extent.

Chapter 4
Tips to Stay on Track

There are some tips that you will have to keep in mind if you do not want to deviate from your diet. These tips can be thought of as tips for achieving success. A couple of tips that are very simple to remember and also are extremely effective would including the reading of labels carefully, look for any carbs that are well hidden, calculate the amount of carbs that you are consuming and also carefully check the serving size according to which the nutritional information is given.

Following are some tips that you might want to keep in mind if you really want to stay on the Atkins bandwagon and not go off tangent.

You need to understand the food products you are consuming

The Atkins diet is all about eating the right products. You will learn about all the foods that are good for you and the food that your body needs to lose the excess weight or to maintain the weight you are at. You should also learn about the foods that will help you cut down on empty carbs that you might be consuming, about foods that have added sugars that you need to avoid. It is all about reading the labels properly and getting a clear understanding of the nutritional facts table given on food products.

Customize your diet

The diet plan that you will have to select will depend upon the weight that you want to shed. There are two basic variations present in this diet, the first one is Atkins 20 and the second one is Atkins 40. In Atkins 20 you can consume Net Carbs worth 20 grams and similarly Atkins 40 you can consume up to 40 grams of Net Carbs every day. Apart from this there are a variety of food products that you are free to consume. And once you do that, stick to the diet.

Keep a track of carbs that you consume

It is essential that you keep a track of the number of carbs that you are consuming on a daily basis while on the diet. You first need to understand what Net Carbs are and then method that is made use of to calculate net carbs. You can also make use of the carb counters that are available online and stick to the list of food products that you can consume.

You don't have to obsess over the portions

If you are following the Atkins diet you needn't worry about the calories you are consuming. Just ensure that you have got your common sense to guide you through. You need to understand that consumption of calories is essential for your well being; obviously if you overeat you will end up slowing down the process of weight loss. But if you consume only a few calories you will end up slowing down the metabolism of your body. When this happens, the process of weight loss will come to an abrupt halt. Women can and should consume between 1500 and 1800 calories per day whereas men should ensure that their calorie intake per day is 1800-2200 calories per day.

Don't starve yourself

It doesn't matter which stage of the diet you are at; you need to eat regularly. Ensure that you are have three proper meals every day and some snacks to keep the hunger at bay. Or depending upon your eating habits you can have four or even five small meals at regular intervals. This will ensure that your blood sugar levels don't drop, your energy levels will stay high and it will keep your appetite under your control. You should eat till you get the feeling of being satisfied; you don't have to stuff yourself. In the coming chapters you can take a look at all the various recipes for snacks, meals and even deserts to ensure that you can eat regularly while still following the diet.

Don't forget to include some protein in all your meals

On a daily basis (taking into consideration breakfast, lunch and dinner and all the other snacks in between) you need to ensure that you are consuming at least 4 to 6 ounces of protein. You can choose the protein you want to eat from all the varied meats that you can safely consume when on an Atkins die. You can have eggs, lean or fatty meat depending upon your preference, any form of poultry; you can even opt for marbled cuts of beef if you fancy it. The option of seafood is always open. Ensure that whenever you are opting for a leaner cut then use plenty of olive oil or any one of the healthy oils in your cooked vegetables and salad dressings.

Naturally fatty food is good

It is true that fatty food tastes much better than non-fatty food. And fatty food fills you up more easily when compared to food that is less in fat. Dietary fat is an important aspect of the Atkins diet and it needs to be given due consideration. Dietary fats are essential to maintain your overall health, but stay away from any form of trans fat. These can make you incredibly sick and go against the Atkins diet.

Say no to added sugar

All the soft drinks and most of the other junk food that you are fond of contains a lot of added sugar. These are not the only products or even forms of added sugar. All the processed and manufactured foods are generally high on carbs and calories but don't really have any nutrients. One alternative to this would to make use of non-caloric sweeteners to sweeten your beverages. You can make use of saccharin or a combination of stevia and sucralose. But make sure that you do not exceed 3 grams of Net Carbs per day.

Eat lots of vegetables

You need to ensure that you are consuming at least 12 to 15 grams of carbohydrates in the form of foundation vegetables on a daily basis. You will need to have at least 5 servings of vegetables on a daily basis. When you consume vegetables you get your daily requirement of fiber. And fiber helps in managing the levels of blood sugar in your body. Not just this but fiber also helps to make you feel full and maintain your weight.

Enjoy what you eat

Enjoy what you eat. The Atkins diet simply concentrates on making you eat healthy and wholesome foods that are absolutely delicious. Most of the diets that exist tend to instill a sense of fear into those who pursue it. You don't have to stock up on expensive pre cooked meals or produce. You can carry on eating the everyday ingredients provided that they are low in carbohydrates; don't contain any added sugars and trans fat. You needn't dread going out for a meal, provided you can choose smartly from the menu you are provided. You can go ahead with this diet even when you are travelling or going out simply. If you don't enjoy what you eat, the diet would unnecessarily seem dreadful.

Keep your body hydrated

You need to keep yourself hydrated to ensure that the electrolyte composition of your body does not get disturbed. That would not be a pleasant physical change. You need to keep drinking lots of water, at least 8 glasses and then some more. Also if you can't do away with your daily cup of tea or coffee then you can consume some. But in moderation and let go of the sugar. You can have healthier versions of tea. You could perhaps opt for green tea or even lemon tea. When your body is sufficiently hydrated your body will start letting go of all the water weight that you hold, not to mention it is very healthy.

Daily supplements will help

When on a diet it will be helpful if you take some supplements daily along with all the healthy wholesome food that you are consuming. Ensure that the daily dose of supplement consists of vitamins, minerals, potassium, magnesium, and calcium. Take some iron supplements if you have an iron deficiency, if not you don't need iron supplements. You will also need some Omega-3 fatty oils; fish oil is a good source of this. Consult your doctor before you start taking any supplements.

Physical activity is always welcome

Physical activities as well as exercise are the most natural way to stay fit and healthy. This is the perfect partner for your diet. You can opt for some brisk walking, swimming or any of the more fun activities such as Zumba or eve yoga. Physical activity is an integral part of the Atkins diet. When you start building muscle you also start burning calories. But it would do you some good if you wait for a few weeks before you get started with any form of regular physical exercise. Give your body some time to get adjusted to the new diet and you can get started with any form of physical activity you are interested. Water aerobics and brisk walking will definitely help you lose weight.

Keep a track of your progress

Keep a track of not just the weight that you have managed to shed, but also the manner in which you have managed to improve your health in. once every week you should measure yourself, at your chest, waist and hips. It would also help you to keep track of your progress if you maintain a food journal. It will help you see the improvement you have had while consuming certain products and also the exercising pattern you followed. This will help you make the necessary changes to meet your fitness and health goals. Getting some baseline tests before the beginning of the diet and then comparing it to the tests you have gotten after at least 3 months of following the diet will definitely leave you feeling pleasantly surprised.

Get support from your friends and family

Your friends and family are and will always be your pillars of strength. Let the people who play a major role in your life know that you have started the diet. It will provide you some help to have people who support you around and also provide you the emotional support you will need to continue with the diet

Plan in advance

If you really want to follow this diet then it is essential that you plan well in advance. You will need to stock up your kitchen with food products that are Atkins compatible. You need to have on hand such products that will help you create a good and nutritious meal. It is likely that you will end up going back to your old habits if you don't have any food options on hand. You can also cook batches of food and freeze it all.

Chapter 5
How to Get Started

So, you have decided to get started on the Atkins diet? Well, congratulations are in order, you have taken the right decision and the Atkins diet will help you get started in the right direction towards a slimmer and a healthier you. Not just that, but it will also help you maintain your health and weight as well. Atkins indeed is a really good way to improve your eating baits, shed some extra kilos and ultimately, feel good about yourself. Before you get started with this diet, take a look at the tips mentioned in this chapter. These tips will help you through your diet in a way that is not just healthy but also facilitate you to reach your health and fitness goals.

Set some goals

Goals are essential for staying motivated. So, before you start going into the nuisances of the Atkins diet, it is essential that you have set some goals for yourself. When you do this, it will provide you something to look forward to achieving. Set goals that are achievable and not unrealistic, and the goals should be healthy and help you concentrate on your overall health while shedding those extra kilos. A positive goal will provide you motivation on those days when you feel like you are going off track.

Understand the working of this diet

Before getting started with a full-blown diet, you need to understand not just the manner in which the diet works but also the results you can expect from the diet after putting in some effort. So, take some time out and understand the workings of the weight loss program. For instance, the Atkins program is divided into various phases and in the first phase you condition your body to shift towards burning fat for generating energy instead of carbohydrates like it has always been doing. When this change starts, that is when the diet has actually begun. The ultimate goal of the first phase it to help you gradually decrease your net carb consumption on a daily basis to not more than 20 grams, this is the level where your body starts to burn fat.

You will need a lot of motivation

It does not matter how you got to know about the Atkins diet, be it through a friend or a post on a community blog, it doesn't matter. You will need to find ways in which you can wholly hold yourself accountable towards the diet and you will need to stay motivated for the entire duration of the diet. Losing weight becomes less of a task that you have got to complete and more enjoyable when you are doing it with and around people who support the goals you have set for the diet and this will provide you with all the motivation that you will need to stick to the diet. A little bit of added motivation will indeed make a lot of difference.

Familiarize yourself with the foods you can consume

Before you get started with the diet it is essential that you go through the list of food items that you are allowed and not allowed to eat. When you know all about the ingredients that you are allowed to consume then it becomes easier when you are looking for recipes about what all you can cook. This book contains various recipes for all the different phases of the Atkins diet, so make sure that you have read through them. And there are some deserts as well that you can whip up in your kitchen.

Don't forget to stay hydrated

Staying hydrated is essential for the success of the Atkins diet like any other diet. During the first phase of the diet it is essential that you consume at least 8 glasses of water and some more. Each glass of water must be around 8 ounces and you have the liberty to replace four of these with other beverages you might fancy like tea, coffee, vegetable broth or chicken broth, or light soups. It is really important that you are keeping your body hydrated during the course of the diet, because this is the only way in which you can avoid getting dehydrated or causing any imbalance in your electrolytes that is very likely to happen when your body gets rid of the water weight during the first stage of this diet.

Don't say no to fats

Against the popular belief that consumption of fats will not help the weight reduction process in any manner, it is essential that you keep consuming healthy fats if you want to lose weight while following the Atkins diet. When you consume the essential dietary fats that are required by your body, it will help in the better absorption of all the nutrients that you might be consuming from various other sources. And an added advantage is that fat makes your food taste much better and you can enjoy your food.

Snack at regular intervals

You need to keep snacking at regular intervals. It is not just important that you have some snacks between your meals while following the Atkins diet, but it is actually encouraged. You can have up to two snacks between breakfast, lunch and dinner, when you do this it will help you fight off the high carb cravings that our body is susceptible to and will also make you feel full. You can avoid overeating in this manner. When you can keep your hunger at bay, only then will you be able to stick with the course of this diet. When the temptation of high carbs has been driven away by delicious low carb snacks, the chances of straying away reduce exponentially. You can look into the delicious snack recipes that are mentioned in this book to keep your hunger in check.

Well, congratulations on having decided to give the Atkins diet a whirl, it is more than a diet it is a lifestyle in itself. You are on the right path towards achieving your weight and fitness goals. These tips can come in handy when you are begging the diet. All the best!

Chapter 6
Some Myths and Facts

One of the popular low carb diets is the Atkins diet and it is believed to increase the rate of weight loss by at least 3 percent, without any additional exercise. Just by following the diet you can shed more than a few kilos. Atkins diet has become a fad in the last couple of years. When anything becomes a fashion and comes into the spotlight, a lot of myths and misconceptions tend to be generated about it. The misconceptions relate to how the diet works or even the basis of the diet. Before you get started with the diet it is essential to put these misconceptions to rest. There have been a number of studies and there have been a fair share of disagreements about the effectiveness of the Atkins diet. All these have lead to the various misconceptions about this diet.

In this chapter we will take a look at some of the most common myths associated with the Atkins diet.

Deficient in nutrients

"It is deficient in nutrients", this perhaps is one of the most common misconceptions one can have about the Atkins diet. This means that people tend to believe that the required amount of vegetables and fruits that one needs to consume to stay healthy are deprived when following the Atkins diet. It is exactly what others perceive it to be, a misconception. This is not a fact, it's a myth. Research shows that individuals who have been on the Atkins diet ended up consuming more fruits and vegetables than they did previously. When you get started with the Atkins diet, the induction phase ensures that the individuals following it need to have at least five servings of fruits and vegetables that are high in nutrients on a daily basis. But the vegetables and fruits that you are consuming need to be low in sugar content. Once you get done with the induction phase you are at a liberty to add more fruits and vegetables as you go along the diet. So, it really isn't logical that the Atkins diet is low in nutrients. Studies show that hardly one third of the population consumes the sufficient 5 servings of fruits and vegetables on a daily basis. So, if you get started with the Atkins diet you will actually start consuming the desired amount of these things.

A low carb diet will tire you easily

A lot of people are of the misconception that when you are following a diet that is low on carbohydrates such as the Atkins diet then you will feel more tired than usual because there are no carbohydrates in it to give you any energy. But in fact when you overload your system with more carbohydrates than it actually requires even then you end up tiring yourself. When you overload your system with unrequited carbs your blood sugar will oscillate between two extremes and this either makes your system hyper or assists in its crash. When you follow the Atkins diet, your body will get a steady supply of carbohydrates that it requires and this will help in maintaining a more balanced level of blood sugar and stabilize your body. Once your blood sugar levels are sufficiently stabilized, you will feel more energetic than usual and even your metabolism will improve. One important hurdle that you will phase while on this diet is the reduction in the natural salt content in your body. When you get rid of all the water weight, you will also get rid of the essential salt in your body, and when this happens you will feel tired because the electrolytes in your body are out of whack. So, it is quintessential that you regularly monitor your sodium level and keep it balanced; any imbalance in it will make you feel really tired. You will not only have to monitor your sodium levels, but you might also have to take a supplement that includes calcium, potassium and magnesium to ensure that the salt levels in the body are normal.

Reduction of only the water weight

This is true in the initial phase of the Atkins diet; your body does get rid of all the water weight. But then again, the same is true for any other diet that exists. Water weight will be the first weight that your body will get rid of when you start a new diet. Only after getting through the initial week of following the Atkins diet will your body actually start burning fat. Once you cut out the supply of carbohydrates to your body or bring it down to a minimal level that is when your body will start burning of the fat for generating energy. Once you have lost the water weight initially the rate at which you shed weight from then on will slow down.

Be prepared to get constipated

This is a quite an odd misconception that if you are on the Atkins diet you will get constipated, because this diet doesn't provide the required fiber intake for your body. It is just a misconception, in fact the diet allows for you to consume foods that are rich in fiber like broccoli, spinach and eggplant. Not just this but you can even consume a lot of leafy greens and even asparagus while on the diet. Once you have pulled through the induction phase of the diet, you can incorporate more fruits and vegetables into your diet and this will help in increasing the fiber content in your diet. All this adds up to making your gut healthy. If you are really worried about it then you can eat a flax meal or take fiber supplements to help with your bowel movement, but this isn't an issue that everyone will have to go through. And this definitely is not something that should keep you from trying out this diet. A lot of people can maintain their bowel movement even when they change their diets, so if you think you might need some little help you can always opt for a flax meal in the initial stages of the diet. Constipation is not really a side effect associated with this diet, you needn't worry about this.

The weight loss is temporary

A lot of people consider the Atkins diet to be effective temporarily and also that the weight loss routine on this diet is not long term in nature. In fact, the truth cannot be more far off from it. The Atkins diet is all about promoting a change to your eating habits that is going to be long term in nature and when you do follow this diet it will not only help you in shedding the extra kilos but it will also help you to keep them at bay, provided you continue to follow the diet. The Atkins diet is divided into four phases and each of these phases lets you consume a little more of carbs than the previous stage in a progressive manner. When you move along the diet it will help you figure out the level of carbs that is suitable for your body, along with this it also helps you consume a more healthy diet and also shed some weight while following the healthy routine. The Atkins diet provides for you to consume a variety of ingredients that are not just healthy but tasty as well. All this variety lets you cook foods that aren't repetitive or monotonous and this will provide you the change you require. All this variety will also help you to want to stick to this diet in the long run.

Susceptible to gallbladder disease

The myth that since the Atkins diet is rich in fat it is the cause for several gallbladder diseases; this is not true and is based on dubious data. Studies show that the reason for gallbladder disease is gallstones and these are proven to occur when the fat levels in the body are very low. So, the reason for gallbladder diseases and associated problems would be not getting sufficient fat in your body and not the presence of too much fat. When you don't consume sufficient fat then it doesn't allow the gallbladder to contract and when this happen biliary statis occurs, this means that the bile salt gets crystallized into stone. The one way in which you can prevent this from happening is by ensuring that your gallbladder stays active. And this happens when you consume fatty food and the myth that Atkins causes gallbladder disease is disproved. As is the case with any other diet, even with the Atkins diet you need to ensure that your body is in harmony. The Atkins diet does not consume only fatty foods and it is not completely devoid of fat, it provides the perfect amount of dietary fat that is required for the proper working of your organs.

Hannah Olson

Chapter 7
Atkins Phase 1 Recipes

American Steak (Dinner):

Ingredients:

- 10 ounce skirt steak

- 1 tablespoon hot chili sauce

- 3 cups baby spinach

- 1 ounce pepper Jack cheese, shredded

- 1 teaspoon canola oil

- 1 teaspoon salt or to taste

Method:

1. Rub the chili sauce all over the steak and keep aside.

2.   Place a nonstick skillet over medium heat. Add oil, when the oil is heated add the steaks. Cook on both the sides until golden brown or the color you desire. When done, remove and keep warm.

3.   To the same skillet, add the baby spinach. Sauté for a couple of minutes until the spinach wilts. Sprinkle salt and add the cheese. Cook for a minute or until the cheese melts.

4.   Transfer on to a serving platter. Place the warm steaks over the spinach and serve immediately.

Thai Chicken (Dinner):

Ingredients:

- ¾ pound chicken breast, skinless, cut into 2-inch pieces

- 1 tablespoons Thai fish sauce

- ½ tablespoons tamari soy sauce

- ½ tablespoon water

- 1 teaspoons granular sugar substitute

- 2 tablespoon peanut oil

- 2 green onions, thinly sliced

- 1 teaspoon garlic, chopped

- Crushed red chili flakes to taste

- ½ cup fresh chopped basil

Method:

1.　　To marinate the chicken: Mix together the chicken, fish sauce, tamari sauce, water and sugar substitute. Keep it aside for 30 minutes.

2.　　Place a skillet over medium heat. Add oil. When oil is heated, add green onions and sauté for a couple of minutes or until soft. Add garlic and red chili flakes and sauté for a few seconds.

3.　　Add only the chicken and stir-fry until the chicken is cooked. Transfer on to a serving platter.

4.　　Meanwhile transfer the marinade into a saucepan. Place the saucepan over low heat and bring to a boil. Simmer for a couple of minutes and remove from heat.

5.　　Add basil. Mix well. Pour the sauce over the chicken and garnish with a few leaves of basil.

Chicken Kiev (Dinner):

Ingredients:

- 2 large chicken breasts, skinless, boneless, tenders removed

- Black pepper powder to taste

- 4 cloves garlic, minced

- 1 tablespoon parsley, finely chopped

- 3 tablespoons refrigerated butter

- 1 small egg, beaten

- 1 tablespoon heavy cream

- ¼ cup pork rinds, finely ground

- ¼ cup parmesan, grated

- Vegetable oil for deep frying

- Lemon wedges to serve

Method:

1. With a meat mallet, pound the chicken breasts until it is about ¼ inch thick. Season one side of the chicken breast with black pepper.

2. Sprinkle garlic and parsley (at the center) over the peppered side of the chicken breasts.

3. Chop the butter into 2 squares. Place over the center of the chicken breasts. Fold over the sides of the chicken over the butter and roll it lengthwise. Butter should be completely inside the rolled chicken. Fasten with mini skewers.

4. Mix eggs and cream together and keep aside.

5. Mix together pork rinds and Parmesan.

6. Now dip the rolled chicken into the egg mixture. Roll into pork rind mixture. Keep in the refrigerator for 10 minutes.

7. Pour oil in a deep skillet. Heat over medium heat. When the oil is hot and almost smoking, add the chicken roll. Fry until golden brown. Flip sides over. Fry the other side to golden brown too.

8.   Remove with a slotted spoon and drain on paper towels.

9.   Remove the mini skewers and place on a serving plate. Serve with lemon wedges.

Zucchini Gratin (Lunch):

Ingredients:

- 4 cups zucchini, sliced

- Pepper powder to taste

- ½ cup parmesan cheese

- 2 tablespoons butter, melted

- Cooking spray

Method:

1.   Microwave the zucchini slices on High for 3 minutes.

2.   Spray a baking dish with cooking spray.

3.   Lay the zucchini slices in the dish overlapping each other. Sprinkle pepper powder. Sprinkle cheese all over.

4.   Place in a preheated oven at 400 degree F for about 30 minutes.

5.   Pour the melted butter all over the cheese. Raise the temperature to 475 degree F and bake until the top is golden brown.

6.   Serve hot.

Asparagus and Leek Soup:

Ingredients:

- 4 tablespoons unsalted butter stick

- 2 leeks, sliced

- 1 1/2 pounds asparagus, chopped

- 2 teaspoons garlic, minced

- 2 cans (14.5 ounce each) vegetable broth or homemade broth

- 2/3 cup heavy cream

Method:

1.   Place a large saucepan or pot over medium heat. Add butter. When the butter melts, add leeks. Sauté for a couple of minutes. Add asparagus and sauté for a minute. Add garlic and sauté until fragrant.

2.   Add vegetable broth and bring to a boil. Reduce heat, cover and simmer for a while until the asparagus is tender.

3.   Add cream, salt and pepper. Cool slightly and blend in a blender until smooth. Alternately you can blend with an immersion blender.

4.   Pour the soup back to the pot and reheat thoroughly. Adjust the seasoning if necessary.

5.   Ladle into individual soup bowls and serve.

Ancho Macho Chili (Lunch):

Ingredients:

- 1 large onion

- 100 ounces steak, boneless

- 4 teaspoons chili powder or to taste

- Black pepper powder to taste

- Salt to taste

- 20 ounces canned tomatoes with green chilies

- 3 teaspoons garlic, minced

- 9 ounces table wine or chicken broth

- 5 tablespoons Extra virgin olive oil

Method:

1. Season beefsteak with salt and pepper and keep aside for 10 minutes.

2. Meanwhile heat a large saucepan or pot over high heat. Add half the oil to it. Add the steak in batches and cook until browned well all over. Remove from the pot and keep aside.

3. Add the remaining oil to the same pot. Add onions. Sauté until light brown. Add garlic and sauté until fragrant.

4. Add chili powder, wine or broth and tomatoes. Mix well. Reduce heat and simmer for a couple of minutes.

5. Add the browned beef along with its juices. Cover and cook until the beef is cooked through. It can take a couple of hours.

Old Fashioned Cole Slaw (Lunch):

Ingredients:

- 1 cup vinegar

- 1 cup whipping cream

- 4 large eggs, lightly beaten

- 1/2 cup Splenda or to taste

- Pinch of salt

- 3 tablespoons butter, cut in pieces

- 4 pounds cabbage, shredded

Method:

1. To make the dressing: Add vinegar, cream, egg, splenda and salt to a heavy bottomed pan.

2. Place the saucepan over low heat. Whisk constantly until thick. Remove from heat. Cool slightly.

3. Add butter and mix until it melts.

4.   Place the cabbage in a large serving dish. Pour the dressing over the cabbage. Toss well.

5.   Refrigerate and serve chilled.

Moroccan Meatballs (Dinner):

Ingredients:

For the meatballs:

- 1/4 cup parsley leaves

- 1/2 tablespoon paprika

- 1 teaspoon ground cumin

- 1/2 teaspoon salt

- 1/4 teaspoon ground black pepper or to taste

- 1 pound ground lamb

For the sauce:

- 1/2 tablespoon coconut oil

- 1 large onion, diced

- 2 cloves garlic, crushed

- 1 teaspoon paprika

- 1 teaspoon ground cumin

- 1/4 teaspoon black pepper

- 1/2 teaspoon salt

- 1 cup tomatoes, diced

- 3/4 cup water

- 1/3 cup tomato paste

- 1/4cup fresh parsley leaves, minced

- 2 tablespoons roasted pistachios, chopped to garnish

Method:

1.   To make the meatballs: Mix together all the ingredients of the meatballs using your hands until well combined.

2.   Using your hands, make small meatballs and place them on a baking sheet.

3.   To make the sauce: Place a skillet over medium heat. Add oil. When the oil is hot, add onions. Sauté until the onions are translucent.

4.   Add garlic, paprika, cumin, salt and pepper. Sauté for about 30-40 seconds.

5.   Add tomatoes, sauté for a minute. Add rest of the ingredients of the sauce and mix well. Bring to boil.

6.   Gently lower the meatballs into the sauce. Lower heat, cover and simmer for about 35-40 minutes.

7.   Garnish with pistachio and serve.

Baby Spinach Omelet (Breakfast):

Ingredients:

- 4 eggs, whisked well

- 2 cups baby spinach, torn

- 3 tablespoons parmesan, grated

- ½ teaspoon onion powder

- ¼ teaspoon ground nutmeg

- Salt to taste

- Pepper powder to taste

- Cooking spray

Method:

1. To the beaten eggs, add spinach, cheese, nutmeg, salt, pepper and onion powder. Mix well.

2. Place a nonstick pan over medium heat. Spray with cooking spray.

3. Pour the egg mixture and cook until almost set and the bottom side is golden brown.

4. Flip sides and cook the other side too.

5. Serve hot.

Cheesy Tuna Casserole (Breakfast):

Ingredients:

- 3 cans (6 ounce each) tuna, drained

- 24 ounces frozen chopped French green beans, cooked according to instructions on the package

- 5 ounces fresh mushrooms, chopped,

- 2 stalks celery, finely chopped

- 3 tablespoons onion, finely chopped

- 3 tablespoons butter

- 3/4 cup chicken broth

- 1 cup heavy cream or more if required

- Salt to taste

- Pepper powder to taste

- Xanthan gum (optional)

- 8 ounces cheddar cheese, shredded

Method:

1.　Place a skillet over medium heat. Add butter. When butter melts, add onions and sauté for a couple of minutes. Add mushrooms and celery and sauté until light brown.

2.　Add broth and boil until the broth reduces in quantity by half. Reduce heat until thick. Stir on and off.

3.　Add salt and pepper to taste. Add tuna, beans and the sautéed mushrooms to a casserole dish. Season with salt and pepper.

4.　Top with cheese.

5.　Bake in a preheated oven at 350 degree F until the cheese is melted and bubbling.

Veggie Fajitas (Lunch):

Ingredients:

- 4 teaspoons olive oil

- 4 cloves garlic, minced

- 2 green bell peppers, sliced

- 2 red bell peppers, sliced

- 2 yellow peppers, sliced

- 2 orange bell peppers, sliced

- 1 onions sliced

- 2 cups mushrooms, sliced

- 6 green onions, chopped

- Lemon pepper to taste

Method:

1. Place a large pan or wok over medium heat. Add olive oil. When oil is hot, add onions and garlic. Sauté for a

couple of minutes. Add bell peppers. Sauté for a couple of minutes.

2.   Add mushrooms and green onions. Sauté until the mushrooms are tender.

3.   Add salt and pepper and mix well and serve.

Cauliflower Mashed Potatoes (Dinner or Lunch):

Ingredients:

- 2 heads cauliflower, chopped into florets

- 1/2 cup sour cream

- 1/4 cup butter, salted

Method:

1. Place the cauliflower in a steamer and steam until soft.

2. Transfer the contents into a large pan and place the pan on high heat to remove the extra moisture.

3. Add the cauliflower to a food processor and process until you get a mashed potato consistency.

4. Add butter and mix well. Add sour cream. Mix well and serve.

Chilled Lemon Cheesecake (Dessert):

Ingredients:

- 2 ounces gelatin powder

- 2 cups water

- 2 pounds cream cheese

- 12 sachets sugar substitute or to taste

- Juice of 2 lemons

- Zest of 2 lemons or to taste

- A large pinch of salt

- Thinly sliced lemon for garnishing

- 1 teaspoon lemon zest, shredded

Method:

1. Add water to a saucepan. Sprinkle gelatin powder all over the water. Keep it aside for about 10 minutes to dissolve.

2.   Meanwhile add cream cheese and sugar substitute to a bowl. Beat until creamy.

3.   Place the saucepan with gelatin over low heat. Stir constantly until the gelatin dissolves. Remove from heat.

4.   Pour the gelatin mixture into the cream cheese mixture and beat well.

5.   Add lemon juice, lemon zest and salt and blend again.

6.   Transfer the beaten mixture into a cake tin. Refrigerate overnight.

7.   Garnish with lemon slices and shredded lemon zest.

Hannah Olson

Chapter 8
Atkins Diet Phase 2 Recipes:

Egg muffins (Breakfast):

Ingredients:

- 10 large eggs, beaten

- 1 medium green bell pepper, diced

- ¾ cup low fat cheddar cheese

- 3 tablespoons feta cheese

- 1 teaspoon garlic seasoning or to taste

Method:

1.   To the beaten eggs, add green pepper and garlic seasoning.

2.   Grease muffin molds. Pour the egg mixture (3/4 full) into the muffin molds.

3.   Bake in a preheated oven at 375 degree F for 25-30 minutes or until the muffins are set and browned.

4.   Serve hot. They can last for a week if refrigerated.

Kebab Platter (Dinner):

Ingredients:

- 7 ounce lamb, cut into 1 ½ inch cubes

- 1 medium eggplant, cut into 1 ½ inch cubes

- 1 red onion, cut into 1 ½ inch cubes

- 1 medium red bell pepper, cut into 1 ½ inch cubes

- Salt to taste

- Pepper powder to taste

- Red chili flakes to taste

- 2 tablespoons lemon juice

- Normal skewers or bamboo skewers

Method:

1.   If you are using the bamboo skewers, soak in warm water for at least 20 minutes

2.   Thread the lamb, eggplant, onion, and pepper pieces on to the skewers. Sprinkle salt, pepper and chili flakes.

3.   Place in a preheated grill and grill until the lamb is cooked. Turn the skewers a couple of times.

4.   Remove from the skewers and sprinkle lemon juice.

Avocado Zucchini Soup:

Ingredients:

- 1 tablespoon extra-virgin olive oil

- 2 green onions, chopped, divided

- 1 teaspoon ginger root, grated

- 1 garlic clove, chopped

- 15 ounce vegetable broth

- ½ cup water

- 1 medium zucchini, thinly sliced

- ¼ teaspoon salt

- Pepper powder to taste

- ½ has avocado, chopped

- 1 tablespoon lemon juice

- 1 tablespoon red bell pepper, chopped

Method:

1.   Place a large saucepan over medium heat. Add olive oil. Leaving aside 1 tablespoon of the green onion, add the rest to the saucepan. Sauté for 2-3 minutes.

2.   Add ginger and garlic. Sauté for a minute. Add vegetable broth, water, zucchini, salt and pepper.

3.   Cover and cook for a while until the zucchini is tender. Remove from heat and let it cool for a while.

4.   Add avocado. Blend the soup in a blender or with a stick blender. Transfer the soup back to the saucepan. Bring to a boil.

5.   Remove from heat. Add lemon juice and red bell pepper. Mix well. Sprinkle the retained green onions.

Blueberry Cooler:

Ingredients:

- 1 cup cucumber, skinned, seeded, chopped

- ¼ cup fresh lemon juice

- ¼ cup fresh or frozen blueberries

- 3 teaspoons granular sugar substitute or to taste

- 2 teaspoons fresh rosemary

- Crushed ice

- 2 ounce gin (optional)

- 6 ounce club soda

Method:

1.   Blend together the cucumber, lemon juice, blueberries, sugar substitute until smooth.

2.   Add rosemary and pulse a couple of times. Strain the blended mixture with a wire mesh strainer.

3.   Pour into glasses (up to ¼ in each glass). Add gin and soda to fill it up.

4.   Stir well. Serve with crushed ice

Atkins Cuisine Bread

Ingredients:

- 2 cups + 1 tablespoon Atkins cuisine all purpose baking mix - refer recipe 11 further down

- 1 1/2 tablespoons baking powder

- 1/2 teaspoon salt

- 1 packet granular sugar substitute

- 18 tablespoons cold water

- 3 tablespoons vegetable oil

Method:

1. Mix together all the dry ingredients in a large bowl.

2. Add water and oil. Use a spatula mix well to form a dough.

3. Take out the dough from the bowl using the spatula and place on a lightly greased, clean surface.

4.   Coat your hands with some oil. Using your hands shape the dough as desired

5.   Place the dough into a greased bread pan.

6.   Bake the bread in a preheated oven at 350 degrees F for 1 hour or until done.

7.   Remove from oven and place on a wire to cool.

8.   Slice only when cooled completely and serve. Store unused bread in an airtight container.

Almond Soy Mini Muffins (Breakfast):

Ingredients:

- 1 cup unsalted butter, softened

- 1 1/2 cups granulated Splenda

- 1 teaspoon vanilla extract

- 6 eggs

- 1 cup ground almond

- 1 cup soy flour

- 6 teaspoons cinnamon powder

- 1 teaspoon baking powder

- 1/2 teaspoon salt

Method:

1. Mix together all the dry ingredients in a large bowl.

2. In another bowl, add butter, vanilla and sweetener. Whip until light and fluffy.

3.   Gradually add eggs one by one and beat well.

4.   Add the dry ingredients, a little at a time and fold gently.

5.   Spoon the batter into lined mini muffin pans (keep it 3/4 full).

6.   Bake in a preheated oven at 355 degree F for about 18-20 minutes or until a toothpick when inserted in the center comes out clean.

Chocolate Soy Pancakes (Breakfast)

Ingredients:

- 2 cups soy flour

- 10 tablespoons granulated splenda or to taste

- 6 tablespoons unsweetened cocoa powder

- 1 teaspoon baking powder

- 1/2 teaspoon salt

- 2 cups milk

- 4 large eggs beaten

- 6 tablespoons unsalted butter, melted

- Cooking spray

Method:

1. Mix together all the dry ingredients in a large bowl.

2. Add milk, eggs and butter and mix until well combined. Keep aside for 5-10 minutes.

3.   Place a nonstick pan over medium heat. Spray with cooking spray. When the pan is heated, add about 1/4 cup of the batter. Spread it a little. Cook until the bottom side is golden brown. Flip sides and cook the other side too. Remove and keep warm.

4.   Repeat step 3 with the remaining batter.

5.   Serve butter.

Spinach and Strawberry Salad (Lunch):

Ingredients:

- 6 cups of spinach, chopped

- 1 1/2 cups of strawberries, sliced

- 3/4 cup slivered almonds

- 1/2 Haas avocado, diced

- 3 tablespoons orange juice

- 3 tablespoons olive oil

- 2 tablespoons balsamic vinegar

- 1 tablespoon Dijon-style prepared mustard

- Salt to taste

- Pepper powder to taste

Method:

1.   To make the dressing: Whisk together orange juice, oil, vinegar, salt, pepper and mustard.

2.   Mix together rest of the ingredients in a bowl.

3.   Pour the dressing. Toss well and serve.

Herb Crusted Salmon (Dinner):

Ingredients:

For the salmon:

- 3 salmon fillets (6 ounces each)

- 2 tablespoons coconut flour

- 3 tablespoons fresh parsley or 3 teaspoons dried

- 1 1/2 tablespoons olive oil

- 1 1/2 tablespoons Dijon mustard

- Salt to taste

- Pepper powder, to taste

For the salad:

- 3 cups arugula

- 1 small red onion, sliced thin

- 3 tablespoons lemon juice

- 1 1/2 tablespoon white wine vinegar

- 1 1/2 tablespoon olive oil

- Salt to taste

- Pepper powder to taste

Method:

1. Mix together olive oil and Dijon. Rub this mixture into the salmon fillets.

2. Place the salmon fillets on a line-baking sheet.

3. Mix together in a small bowl, coconut flour, parsley, salt and pepper. Sprinkle this mixture over the salmon.

4. Bake in a preheated oven at 450 degree F for about 10-15 minutes or until cooked.

5. Meanwhile, mix together all the salad ingredients in a bowl. Toss well.

6. To serve: Place salad on individual plates. Top each plate with salmon and serve.

Lobster Salad (Salad):

Ingredients:

- 1 1/2 pounds Northern lobster

- 4 cup Chinese cabbage (Bok-Choy or Pak-Choi), shredded

- 1 small red peppers

- 8 medium spring onions

- 2 tablespoons sesame seeds

- Salt to taste

- Pepper powder to taste

For dressing:

- 4 tablespoons rice vinegar

- 4 tablespoons tamari sauce

- 2 tablespoons canola oil

- 2 teaspoons sesame oil

- 2 teaspoons ginger, minced

Method:

1.   To make the dressing: Mix together all the ingredients of the dressing in a bowl. Whisk well.

2.   Mix together rest of the ingredients in a large bowl. Pour the dressing over the salad. Toss well and serve.

All Purpose Low Carb Baking Mix:

Ingredients:

- 1/2 cup crude wheat bran

- 10 ounces vanilla whey protein powder

- 10 ounces vital wheat gluten

- 2 1/4 cups whole grain soy flour

- 1/2 cup whole ground golden flaxseed meal

Method:

1.   Mix together all the ingredients and store in an airtight container. Refrigerate until use. It can store up to a month.

Asian Beef Salad with Edamame (Lunch):

Ingredients:

- 2 scallions or spring onions

- 1/2 teaspoon garlic, minced

- 1 tablespoon tamari sauce

- 1/2 teaspoon rice vinegar

- 1/2 teaspoon toasted sesame oil

- 1/4 teaspoon splenda

- 9 ounces beef top sirloin, trimmed of fat

- 1/4 teaspoon curry powder

- 1 teaspoon ginger, ground

- 1 tablespoon canola oil

- 1 1/2 cups spring mix salad

- 1 small red bell pepper, chopped into strips

- 4 ounces water chestnuts

- 1 cup shelled edamame

Method:

1.   Add to a bowl, green onions, garlic, tamari sauce, rice vinegar, sesame oil, and splenda. Mix well.

2.   Pour half of this into a zip lock plastic bag. Keep the remaining half aside.

3.   To the zip lock bag, add steak and marinate for 7-8 hours in the refrigerator.

4.   Place a large skillet over high heat. Add canola oil. When the oil is very hot, remove beef from the zip lock bag and add to the skillet. Fry for 2-4 minutes until the beef is cooked. Transfer into a large serving bowl.

5.   Add mixed greens, bell pepper, water chestnuts, and edamame and mix well.

6.   To the other half of the sauce that was kept aside, add curry powder and ginger.

7.   Pour this over the salad. Toss well and serve.

Steamed Cinnamon Coconut Milk Egg Custard (Dessert):

Ingredients:

- 4 eggs

- 4 egg yolks

- 2/3 cup granulated sweetener like splenda

- 4 cups unsweetened coconut milk

- ½ teaspoon ground cinnamon

- 1/2 tsp salt

Method:

1. Whisk together eggs and egg yolks in a bowl. Add sweetener and mix well.

2. To another bowl add coconut milk, cinnamon and salt. Whisk well.

3. Pour the coconut milk mixture into the egg yolk mixture. Whisk well.

4.   Pour into greased ramekins.

5.   Place a baking tray with water in it in a preheated oven. Place the ramekins into a baking tray, which is filled with water.

6.   Bake in a preheated oven at 300 degree F for about 30 minutes or until the custard is set.

7.   Serve either warm or cold.

Kale Salad (Lunch):

Ingredients:

- 1 head kale

- 2 cups mixed greens

- 2 cucumbers, peeled and diced

- 4 avocados, peeled, pitted, diced

- 4 tomatoes, diced

- 2 cans garbanzo beans (chickpeas), drained and rinsed

Topping:

- Hemp seeds or sunflower seeds

Dressing:

- 1 cup tahini

- 1 1/2 cups water + more if required

- ¼ cup lemon juice

- 2 cloves garlic, minced

- Salt to taste

- Pepper powder, to taste

Method:

1.   To make the dressing: Add all ingredients of the dressing to a bowl. Whisk well.

2.   Add the salad ingredients to a bowl. Pour the dressing over it. Mix well.

3.   Refrigerate for 3-4 hours before serving.

Chapter 9
Atkins Diet Phase 3 Recipes

Cheddar Cheese Open Sandwiches (any meal):

Ingredients:

- 2 tablespoons olive oil

- 1 medium red onion, thinly sliced

- 2 tablespoons balsamic vinegar

- 1 teaspoon granular sugar substitute (sucralose)

- 8 ounce sharp cheddar, thinly sliced

- Salt to taste

- Pepper to taste

- 8 slices Atkins cuisine bread

Method:

1.   Place a skillet over medium heat. Add oil. When oil is heated add onions. Sauté until the onions are light brown.

2.   Add balsamic vinegar, sugar substitute, salt and pepper. Mix well.

3.   Toast the bread lightly. Lay the cheese slices over the bread. Divide the onion mixture over the cheese. Spread well.

4.   Place in a preheated broiler 4 inches from the heat source and broil until the cheese melts. Serve hot.

French Onion Soup:

Ingredients:

- ½ cup butter

- 7 cups leeks

- 2 tablespoons stevia or to taste

- 7 cups stock (vegetable or beef or chicken)

- ¼ cup dry white wine

- 4 cloves garlic, crushed

- ¼ teaspoon thyme

- Salt to taste

- Pepper powder to taste

- 1 dozen pork rinds, crumbled

- ¼ cup parmesan, grated

- ½ cup cheese of your choice

Method:

1.   Place a skillet over medium heat. Add butter. When the butter melts, add leeks. Sauté for 3-4 minutes.

2.   Lower heat and cover. Cook for about 9-10 minutes. Stir a couple of times.

3.   Raise the heat to high. Add garlic and stevia. Sauté for a couple of minutes. Stir constantly.

4.   Add broth, white wine, thyme, salt and pepper. Bring to a boil. Simmer for about 15 minutes.

5.   Transfer the soup into ovenproof bowls. Sprinkle the pork rinds, cheese, and Parmesan over the soup.

6.   Place in a preheated broiler and broil until the cheese is slight brown.

7.   Serve hot.

Strawberry Shake (Breakfast):

Ingredients:

- 2 glasses of water

- 2 scoops whey protein powder

- 2 teaspoons bee pollen

- 15 -20 frozen strawberries

Method:

1.   Blend together all the ingredients until smooth. Transfer into tall glasses. Serve with crushed ice.

Zucchini Bread:

Ingredients:

- 2 cups almonds, finely ground

- 2 cups soy flour

- 2 cups granular sugar substitute

- 3 teaspoons ground cinnamon

- 1 teaspoon ground nutmeg

- 1 teaspoon salt

- 1 teaspoon baking soda

- 1 teaspoon baking powder

- 1 cup canola oil

- 8 large eggs

- 2 medium zucchini, grated

- 2 teaspoons vanilla extract

Method:

1.   Mix together all the dry ingredients in a large bowl.

2.   In another bowl, add eggs, oil, zucchini, and vanilla extract. Whisk well. Pour this mixture into the dry mixture bowl. Mix well until the batter is well combined.

3.   Transfer the batter into a generously greased bread pan.

4.   Place the pan in a preheated oven at 350 degree F. Bake for about 45 minutes or until a toothpick when inserted comes out clean.

5.   Remove from the oven. Cool for 10 minutes and remove from the pan.

6.   Cool slightly more and slice into as thick slices as you desire.

Pineapple Almond Milk Smoothie (any time):

Ingredients:

- 40 whole almonds, blanched

- Ice cubes as required

- 5 ounces fresh pineapple, diced, frozen

- 1 cup Greek yogurt

- 1 cup unsweetened almond milk

- 4 sachets sweetener of your choice or to taste

Method:

1. To blanch almonds: Place the almonds in a small saucepan filled with water. Bring to a boil. Simmer for a minute. Drain and rinse with cold water. Remove the skin.

2. Blend together all the ingredients until smooth.

3. Serve in tall glasses garnished with slivered almonds.

Spicy Broiled Orange Chicken Breasts (Dinner):

Ingredients:

- 3 pounds chicken breast, skinless, quartered

- Salt to taste

- Ground black pepper to taste

For marinating

- 1/2 cup fresh orange juice

- 4 teaspoons garlic, finely chopped

- 2 tablespoons olive oil

- 2 tablespoons chili powder or to taste

- 2 teaspoons Splenda sweetener

- 2 teaspoons orange rind, grated

- Cayenne pepper to taste

Method:

1. Sprinkle salt and pepper over the chicken.

2.   Mix together all the ingredients of the marinade. Add chicken pieces. Mix well.

3.   Transfer the entire contents to a large zip lock plastic bag. Refrigerate for a minimum of 8-7 hours.

4.   Preheat a broiler Place the broiler racks such that it is about 6 inches away from the heating element.

5.   Remove from the refrigerator about 30 minutes before broiling.

6.   Broil the chicken for about 12-15 minutes or until done. Turn the chicken once in between.

Mixed Berries Orange Sherbet (any time drink):

Ingredients:

- 1 1/2 cups frozen strawberries

- 1 1/2 cups frozen raspberries

- 1 1/2 cups frozen blueberries

- 2/3 cup granulated sweetener

- Zest of an orange rind, grated

- 1/4 cup water

- 2 cups low-fat buttermilk

Method:

1.   Place berries, sweetener, orange zest and water in a saucepan. Place the pan over medium heat and bring to a boil.

2.   Reduce heat, cover and simmer until the berries have disintegrated. Remove from heat and cool completely.

3.   Blend the berries in a blender until smooth. Strain and keep the puree.

4.   Add buttermilk to the puree and blend it once again until well combined.

5.   Refrigerate for 3-4 hours.

6.   Stir before serving.

Low Carb Whole Grain Pie Crust:

Ingredients:

- 2/3 cup whole-wheat flour

- 2/3 cup soy flour

- 3 ounces vital wheat gluten flour

- 6 tablespoons wheat bran

- 1 teaspoon salt

- 16 tablespoons unsalted cold butter, chopped into small cubes

- 2 tablespoons cold water

Method:

1. Add all the ingredients except cold water to a food processor. Pulse until you get a coarse consistency.

2. With the food processor running, slowly pour the cold water. Pulse until a dough is formed.

3.   Divide the dough into 2 and wrap each in a plastic and freeze for 15 minutes.

4.   Remove from the freezer. Place the dough in between 2 plastic sheets and roll into a 12-inch circular shape.

5.   Place the rolled dough in a 9-inch pie dish such that the sides are also covered. Press the dough on the sides as well as the bottom. Remove the extra dough if any.

6.   Prick the pie with a fork all over.

7.   Bake in a preheated oven at 400 degree F for about 15 - 20 minutes until golden brown.

8.   Remove from the oven and cool on a wire rack. Use as desired.

9.   With the excess dough, which was removed, you can make mini piecrusts with it.

Fruit Salad (Dessert):

Ingredients:

- 2 mangoes, peeled, seeded, diced

- 4 pints strawberries, sliced in half

- 2 pints blueberries

- 5 kiwis, peeled, sliced

- 2 pints raspberries

- 4 peaches, diced

- 1 ounce of triple sec

- Juice of 2 lemons

- Juice of 2 oranges

- 1/4 cup mint leaves, for garnish

Method:

1.   Add all the ingredients to a large bowl. Toss well. Refrigerate and serve chilled garnished with mint leaves.

Asian Vegetable Soup:

Ingredients:

- 1 1/2 cups green onions, chopped

- 1 cup mushrooms, chopped

- 2 tablespoons tamari sauce

- 1 1/2 tablespoons ginger, minced

- 1 clove garlic, minced

- 1 Serrano pepper, chopped

- 1/2 cup tomatoes, chopped

- 3 ounces firm silken tofu

- 1 medium carrot, peeled, chopped

- 2 tablespoons cilantro, chopped

- 1 cup Chinese cabbage (bok choy) shredded

- 3 cups broth (chicken or vegetable)

Method:

1.   Place a saucepan over medium heat. Add broth and tamari and bring to a boil.

2.   Lower heat and add mushrooms, bok choy, ginger and garlic with the chili. Allow it to Simmer until the bok choy tender.

3.   Add tomatoes and green onions with the tofu and carrots. Simmer for a couple of minutes until the greens are wilted.

4.   Add cilantro, mix well and serve immediately.

Mexican Quinoa Casserole:

Ingredients:

- 1/2 tablespoon vegetable oil

- 1 medium onion, chopped

- 1 clove garlic, minced

- 1/2 cup uncooked quinoa

- 14 ounce canned, diced tomatoes, with liquid

- 1/4 cup water

- 1 tablespoon nutritional yeast (optional)

- 1/2 tablespoon tomato paste or ketchup

- 1/2 teaspoon ground cumin

- 1/2 teaspoon oregano

- 1/4 teaspoon chili powder or to taste

- Salt to taste

- Freshly ground pepper powder to taste

- 9 1/2 ounces canned black beans, rinsed, drained

- 5 1/2 ounces canned corn kernels, with liquid

- 2 cups baby spinach

- Cheese to serve

- Cilantro to garnish

Method:

1.   Place a stovetop casserole dish over medium heat. If you don't have one, then place a frying pan. Add olive oil. When the oil is heated, add onions and garlic. Sauté for a while until the onions are translucent. Remove from heat (If you are using frying pan, then transfer the onions to an oven proof dish)

2.   Add quinoa, tomatoes, water, nutritional yeast, tomato paste, cumin, chili powder, oregano, salt and pepper.

3.   Place in a preheated oven at 350 degree F for 30minutes.

4.   Remove the casserole and add spinach. Mix well.

5.   Sprinkle cheese over it and broil for a couple of minutes until the cheese melts.

6.   Garnish with cilantro and serve.

Carrot Edamame salad (Lunch):

Ingredients:

For Salad:

- 10 medium carrots peeled, cut into matchsticks

- 2 cups frozen shelled edamame, thawed

- 1/2 cup black sesame seeds

- ½ cup fresh cilantro, chopped

- Salt to taste

- Pepper powder to taste

- 1 ripe avocado, peeled, pitted chopped

For dressing:

- ½ cup fresh orange juice

- Juice of 2 lime

- Salt to taste

- Pepper powder to taste

- 3 tablespoons agave nectar or raw honey

- 2 inches piece fresh ginger, peeled, grated finely

- 10 drops toasted sesame oil

- ¼ cup grape seed oil

Method:

1.　Mix together all the ingredients of the salad except avocado in a large serving bowl.

2.　To make the dressing: In another bowl, mix together the ginger, lime juice, orange juice, agave nectar salt and pepper, and sesame oil. Whisk well. Whisking constantly, pour the grape seed oil in a thin stream. Whisk until you get a uniform smooth consistency.

3.　To serve: Add the dressing to the salad. Toss well.

4.　Garnish with avocado and cilantro.

Chapter 10
Atkins Diet Phase 4 Recipes

Mexican Strata (Dinner):

Ingredients:

- 10 slices low-carbohydrate bread (Atkins cuisine bread), cubed

- 12 ounces ground turkey sausage

- 6 egg whites

- 2 whole eggs

- 2 cups skim milk

- 1 reduced fat sour cream

- 2 cups cheddar cheese, shredded

- 1/2. Salsa or as desired

- Cooking spray

Method:

1.   Place a skillet over medium heat. Add sausages and cook until browned well.   While cooking, break the sausages.

2.   Grease a pie dish with cooking spray. Place the bread evenly in the dish.

3.   Spread the broken sausages over the bread cubes.

4.   Whisk together in a bowl, whites, eggs, milk and sour cream. Add cheese.

5.   Pour this mixture over the sausages. Cover and place in the refrigerator for a couple of hours.

6.   Remove from the refrigerator and bake in a preheated oven at 325 degree F for about 30 minutes or until light brown on the edges.

7.   Remove from the oven and let cool for 10 minutes before serving.

8.   Serve with salsa

Herb Roasted Vegetables (Dinner):

Ingredients:

- 3 medium sweet potatoes, cut into 1" cubes

- 3 carrots, peeled and cut into 1" pieces

- 2 medium parsnip, peeled and cut into 1" pieces

- 2 small red onion, sliced

- 1 1/2 tablespoons olive oil

- 5 cloves garlic, minced

- 3 teaspoons oregano

- 3 teaspoons thyme

- 3 teaspoons basil

- 1 teaspoon salt

- 1 teaspoon ground black pepper

Method:

1.   Grease a baking dish and place the carrots, sweet potatoes, onions and parsnip in it.

2.   Mix together in a small bowl, garlic, oregano, thyme, basil, salt and pepper and pour over the vegetables. Toss well.

3.   Cover with foil and bake at 425 degree F until tender.

4.   Remove the foil and bake for further 10 minutes.

Calabacitas (Lunch):

Ingredients:

- 3 tablespoon canola oil

- 1 large onion, chopped

- 1 fresh jalapeno pepper, chopped

- 3 pounds zucchini, cut in half lengthwise and then slice

- 1/2 cup corn kernels

- Salt to taste

- 1/2 teaspoon chili powder or to taste

Method:

1.   Place a nonstick skillet over medium heat. Add oil. When oil is hot, add onion and pepper. Sauté until the onion is translucent.

2.   Add zucchini, corn, and salt and chili powder and sauté until the zucchini is soft. Add 3 tablespoons water, cover, and cook for a couple of minutes.

3.   Serve hot.

Pancakes with Turkey sausages (Breakfast):

Ingredients:

- 2/3 cup All Purpose Low-Carb Baking Mix

- 2/3 packet granular sugar substitute (sucralose)

- 1 1/4 teaspoon baking powder

- 1/4 teaspoon salt

- 2/3 cup half and half

- 1 small egg

- 1 cup fresh mango,

- 12 ounces turkey sausage

- Cooking spray

Method:

1.   Mix together all the dry ingredients in a large bowl.

2.   Add egg and half and half. Whisk into a smooth batter. Keep aside for 10 minutes.

3.   Place a nonstick pan over medium heat. Spray with cooking spray.

4.   Make small pancakes. Cook until the bottom side is golden brown. Flip sides and cook the other side too. Remove the pancake and keep warm.

5.   Make pancakes with the remaining batter.

6.   To the same pan, add turkey sausages. Cook until browned well.

7.   Serve with mangoes and sausages.

Chicken Kebabs (Dinner):

Ingredients:

For the Kebabs:

- 6 chicken fillets, de skinned, cut into chunks

- 1/2 cup low carbohydrate yogurt

- 3 teaspoons ginger paste

- 1/2 teaspoon ground turmeric

- 1/2teaspoon ground coriander

- 1/2 teaspoon ground cumin

- Salt to taste

- Freshly ground pepper to taste

For the Dip:

- 1/3 cup crunchy peanut butter

- 3 tablespoons soy sauce

- 3 tablespoons lime juice

- 1 1/2 teaspoon curry paste

- 1/2 cup low carbohydrate yogurt

Method:

1.   Mix together all the ingredients of the kebab except chicken and mix well. Add chicken. Coat the chicken with the marinade.

2.   Thread the chicken kebabs on skewers and grill in a preheated grill for about 10 minutes or until the chicken is cooked.

3.   To make the dip: Add all the ingredients of the dip to a blender. Blend until all the ingredients until smooth.

4.   Garnish the kebabs with shredded cabbage, onion rings and lemon wedges. Serve the kebabs with the dip.

Garlic Potatoes (Dinner):

Ingredients:

- 12 medium sized red or Yukon gold potatoes, rinsed, chopped into small cubes with skin on

- 1/4 cup olive oil

- 1 cup soy or almond milk

- Salt to taste

- Pepper powder to taste

- 5 cloves garlic, minced

- 1/3 cup nutritional yeast (optional)

Method:

1. Place the potatoes in a large saucepan filled with water. Place the saucepan over high heat and bring to a boil. Cook until the potatoes are tender. Drain the water and place the potatoes in a large bowl.

2.   Add rest of the ingredients and mash well and serve with Atkins bread.

Borlotti bean and Kale Soup:

Ingredients:

- 1 ½ tablespoon olive oil

- 1 medium onion, peeled, diced

- 1 large carrot, peeled, diced

- 1 large potato, cut into small chunks

- 1 1/2 tablespoons tomato puree

- A few sprigs fresh thyme

- 1 bay leaf

- 3 cups hot vegetable stock

- 300 g canned borlotti beans, drained, rinsed

- 1/2 bunch curly kale, chopped

- Salt to taste

- Pepper powder to taste

- Parmesan, shredded (optional)

- Crusty bread (optional)

Method:

1. Place a pan over medium heat. Add oil. When oil is hot, add onions and carrots and sauté for 3-4 minutes until the onions are translucent.

2. Add potato, tomato puree, thyme, and bay leaf. Sauté for a couple of minutes and add the stock.

3. Bring to a boil. Lower the heat and simmer for about 10 minutes, covering the pan partially.

4. Add beans, salt, and pepper. Mix well

5. Increase the heat back to medium and bring the soup to a boil.

6. Add kale on top, cook for 5 minutes.

7. Ladle into individual serving bowls, sprinkle Parmesan and serve with crusty bread.

Pineapple Mango Layer Cake (Dessert):

Ingredients:

- 2 cups soy flour

- 2 teaspoons baking powder

- 1/2 teaspoon salt

- 12 large eggs, separated

- 26 tablespoons granular sugar substitute (sucralose), divided

- 4 teaspoons almond extract

- 1/2 cup unsalted butter, melted and cooled

- 1 cup heavy cream

- 1 pineapple, peeled, cored, thinly slice half the pineapple and chop the other half into small pieces

- 1 mango, thinly slice half the mango and chop the other half into small pieces

Method:

1.   To make the cake: Mix together soy flour, baking powder and salt in a bowl.

2.   Whisk the whites using an electric mixer (keep the speed medium) for a couple of minutes.

3.   Add 24 tablespoons of the sugar substitute slowly, beating simultaneously until stiff peaks are formed.

4.   To another bowl add yolks, almond extract and butter. Whisk well.

5.   With the mixer running, gently pour the yolk mixture into the white mixture. Whisk until well combined. Stop the electric mixer now.

6.   Gently fold the flour mixture into the egg mixture.

7.   Divide the batter amongst 2 greased baking dishes.

8.   Bake in a preheated oven at 350 degree F for about 30 minutes or until a toothpick when inserted comes out clean.

9.   Remove from the oven and keep aside to cool for a while. Transfer on to a wire rack to cool completely.

10.   To arrange the cake: Add cream and 2 tablespoons sugar substitute to a bowl and whisk well with an electric mixer until soft peaks are formed.

11.   Place one of the cakes on a plate. Spoon half the whipped cream over it. Spread it all over the cake.

12.   Scatter the mango and pineapple pieces all over the cake.

13.   Place the other cake over the mango and pineapple layer. Spread the remaining whipped cream all over the top of the cake.

14.   Decorate with sliced mangoes and pineapple.

15.   Slice and serve.

Hannah Olson

Chapter 11
Atkins Diet Snacks Recipes

Zucchini Chips:

Ingredients:

- 3 medium zucchini, cut into ¼ inch thick round slices

- 3 tablespoons extra virgin olive oil

- 1/4 teaspoon salt or to taste

- 1/4 black pepper powder

- 1/2 teaspoon paprika

- Garlic powder (optional)

- Any dried herbs like rosemary or dill (optional)

Method:

1. Brush the zucchini slices on both sides with olive oil. Place the zucchini slices on a lined baking sheet.

2. Sprinkle salt, pepper, paprika and herbs, garlic powder if you are using

3. Lay the zucchini slices in a single layer.

4. Bake in a preheated oven at 400 degree F for 10 minutes or until crisp. Turn the chips once half way through.

5. Remove from the oven. Cool on a wire rack and serve.

Note: You can similarly make chips with kale or parsnips.

Salted Crispy Almonds:

Ingredients:

- 2 pounds raw almonds

- 2 tablespoons sea salt

- 1 teaspoon chili powder

- Filtered water

Method:

1. Place the almonds in a bowl. Add water such that the almonds are totally soaked in it. Add salt and mix well. Leave overnight.

2. Drain the water and sprinkle more salt over the almonds. Sprinkle chili powder.

3. Roast in a preheated oven at 170 degree F for a couple of hours until the almonds are crispy.

4. Turn the almonds around a couple of times in between.

5.   Store it in an airtight container.

Note: You can use any types of nuts

Deviled Eggs:

Ingredients:

- 9 eggs, hard boiled, peeled, halved

- 1/2 cup mayonnaise

- 2 teaspoons mustard

- 2 teaspoons ground cumin

- 5 slices bacon

- ¼ teaspoon paprika or to taste

- Sea salt to taste

- Black pepper powder to taste

- Any herbs or seasoning of your choice

Method:

1. Place a nonstick pan over medium heat, Place the bacon slices and cook until crispy.

2. Cool and crumble the bacon.

3.   Scoop out the yolks from then eggs and keep it in a bowl. Mash it.

4.   Add the rest of the ingredients and mix well. Fill the yolk cavities with this filling.

5.   Sprinkle paprika and herbs.

Note: You can use any other filling in it. For example: Instead of bacon you can use avocado. The choice is yours.

Pizza Bites:

Ingredients:

- 3 ounce large pepperoni

- Pizza sauce as required

- Grated cheese as required (optional)

Topping:

- Few olives

- 1/2 green bell pepper, diced

- 1/2 red bell pepper, diced

- 3-4 mushrooms, chopped

- 1/2 cup tomatoes, chopped

Method:

1. Place the pepperoni slices on a lined baking sheet. Bake in a preheated oven at 400 degree F for about 7-8 minutes until the pepperoni is crisp.

2. Spread pizza sauce over each of the pepperoni. Sprinkle mushrooms, bell peppers, tomatoes and cheese.

3. Bake for a few minutes until the cheese melts.

4. Serve immediately.

Note: You can change the toppings and add what you like

Strawberry Mousse (Dessert):

Ingredients:

- 4 ounces fresh strawberries, rinsed, sliced

- 6 tablespoons splenda or 2 tablespoons honey or stevia to taste

- 1/2 tablespoon lemon juice

- 1/4 teaspoon lemon zest, grated

- A pinch salt

- 1 teaspoon unflavored gelatin powder

- 1/2 cup heavy cream

- 1/4 teaspoon vanilla extract

Method:

1. To a small bowl add 2 teaspoons water and gelatin. Keep aside for a while.

2. Meanwhile, blend together strawberries, zest, juice and salt. Transfer the pureed strawberries to a saucepan.

3.   Place the saucepan over medium heat. Add sweetener and heat it slightly (more than warm). Add gelatin mixture. Mix well. Remove from heat.

4.   Keep aside to cool.

5.   Meanwhile whip the cream so as to form soft peaks. Add vanilla and stevia or honey.

6.   Mix well. Add strawberry mixture and fold it gently. Spoon into individual serving bowls.

7.   Chill in the refrigerator. Garnish with strawberry slices and serve.

Veggie Surprise (Dinner):

Ingredients:

- 4 potatoes, peeled, rinsed, diced into 1" cubes

- 6 large carrots, peeled, chopped into chunks

- 4 leeks, green and white parts diced

- 2 pounds Brussels sprouts, halved

- 2 pounds button mushrooms, halved

- 2 heads broccoli, in florets

- 2/3 cup olive oil

- 1/2 cup truffle oil

- 2 tablespoons herbes de Provence

- Salt to taste

- Pepper powder to taste

Method:

1.   Add all the ingredients to an ovenproof dish. Toss well.

2.   Bake in a preheated oven at 400 degree F for about an hour or until the vegetables are tender. Stir the vegetables in between a couple of times.

Quinoa Curry (Dinner):

Ingredients:

- 1/2 cup quinoa, rinsed, drained

- ½ a 400 ml can coconut milk

- ½ a can diced tomatoes

- 1 ½ tablespoons curry powder or to taste

- 2 tablespoons ketchup or tomato paste

- 1 tablespoon coconut oil

- 1 medium onion, chopped

- 1 clove garlic, minced

- 1 medium carrot, peeled, diced

- ½ a 400 gram can chickpeas, drained

- 1 large handful spinach or kale, chopped

- ½ teaspoon crushed red chili pepper

- Salt to taste

- Pepper powder to taste

- Fresh cilantro to garnish

Method:

1. Place a saucepan over medium heat. Add quinoa, coconut milk, and tomatoes with its juice, curry powder and ketchup. Mix well and bring to a boil.

2. Reduce heat, cover and simmer until the quinoa is cooked.

3. Meanwhile, place a pan over medium heat. Add pol. When the oil is hot, add onions and garlic. Sauté until the onions are translucent.

4. Add carrots and chickpeas and cook for 2-3 minutes. Cook for a few minutes.

5. Add spinach and simmer until the spinach wilts. Add quinoa, salt, pepper, red chili pepper, and mix well and remove from heat.

6. Serve garnished with cilantro.

Conclusion

This book covers everything you need to know about the Atkins Diet. The benefits of the diet are immeasurable. You can always use this diet to lose weight but to also keep your immune system stronger. You will be able to avoid many of the diseases and infections that the people of our time are exposed to. You may wonder how you will be able to stick to this diet when you are living in such a fast paced world. But do not worry. This book makes your life easier. You will find a grocery list that will help you finish shopping for the food in this diet in an hour's time!

There are different recipes that have been provided in this book. These recipes cater to the needs of the diet. You will find that most of the food in this diet has very low amounts of sugar and carbohydrates. This is because of the objective of the diet. These recipes leave your mouth watering! I hope you enjoy the different recipes that have been provided for you in this book.

Thank you once again for purchasing the book. I hope you enjoyed reading it!